FERMENTED DELIGHTS

*Unlocking Gut Health
Through Flavor*

Helgalie Suh

Table Of Contents

Chapter 1: The Science of Fermentation

Understanding Fermentation

Fermentation is a natural metabolic process that transforms carbohydrates, such as sugars and starches, into alcohol or organic acids using microorganisms like bacteria, yeast, or fungi. This ancient technique has been utilized for thousands of years, not only as a means of preserving food but also as a way to enhance flavor and nutritional value. The process begins with the introduction of these microorganisms to food, where they thrive in anaerobic environments, breaking down sugars and producing byproducts that contribute to the unique taste and texture of fermented products. Understanding the science behind fermentation allows food lovers to appreciate the complexity and depth of flavors it brings to various dishes. One of the most significant benefits of fermentation is its impact on gut health. Fermented foods are rich in probiotics, live bacteria that can provide health benefits when consumed in adequate amounts. These probiotics help maintain a healthy balance of gut flora, which is essential for digestion, nutrient absorption, and immune function.

The fermentation process also increases the bioavailability of certain nutrients, making them easier for the body to absorb. This includes vitamins such as B12 and K2, as well as minerals like calcium and magnesium. For food lovers, incorporating fermented items into their diets not only enhances flavor but also supports overall health.

Food pairing is another essential aspect of enjoying fermented foods, as certain flavors and textures can complement or enhance one another. Understanding how to pair fermented ingredients with various dishes can elevate meals to new heights. For instance, the tanginess of sauerkraut can brighten a rich, fatty dish like pork belly, while the creaminess of yogurt can balance spicy flavors in Indian cuisine. Additionally, fermented beverages like kombucha or kefir can serve as refreshing accompaniments to meals, further enhancing the overall dining experience. By experimenting with different pairings, food enthusiasts can discover new flavor profiles and maximize the health benefits of their meals. Cooking for specific dietary needs can also be enriched by the versatility of fermented foods. Many individuals have embraced gluten-free, vegan, or dairy-free diets for health or ethical reasons, and fermentation offers a way to create satisfying dishes that meet these requirements. For example, nut-based yogurts can provide the probiotic benefits of traditional dairy yogurt, while fermented vegetables can be used as toppings or side dishes that add depth to plant-based meals.

By exploring fermentation, food lovers can find innovative solutions to dietary restrictions, ensuring that flavor and nutrition are never compromised.

In conclusion, understanding fermentation opens up a world of culinary possibilities for food lovers. The process not only enhances flavors but also contributes to gut health and nutritional density. By embracing fermented foods and exploring their potential in food pairing and dietary adaptations, individuals can create delicious, healthful meals that satisfy both the palate and the body. As interest in fermentation continues to grow, so too does the opportunity to enjoy the myriad benefits it offers in everyday cooking. The Role of Probiotics in Gut Health Probiotics are live microorganisms, often referred to as "good" bacteria, that play a crucial role in maintaining gut health. These beneficial microbes are found in various fermented foods such as yogurt, kefir, sauerkraut, and kimchi. When consumed, probiotics can help balance the gut microbiota, which is essential for digestion, absorption of nutrients, and overall immune function. By incorporating probiotics into the diet, food lovers can enhance their culinary experiences while simultaneously promoting better gut health.

The gut microbiome is a complex ecosystem of trillions of microorganisms that reside in the digestive tract. A healthy balance of these microbes is vital, as an imbalance can lead to issues such as bloating, constipation, and even more serious gastrointestinal disorders. Probiotics contribute to this balance by outcompeting harmful bacteria, producing beneficial compounds, and supporting the integrity of the gut lining. This symbiotic relationship between food and gut health highlights the importance of choosing fermented products as part of a holistic dietary approach. In addition to their role in gut health, probiotics have also been linked to numerous other health benefits. Research suggests that they can aid in reducing inflammation, enhancing mood, and even improving skin conditions. For food enthusiasts, this presents an exciting opportunity to explore diverse fermented foods that not only tantalize the taste buds but also provide significant health advantages. Pairing these foods with prebiotic-rich ingredients, such as garlic, onions, and bananas, can further enhance their effects, creating a delightful synergy that maximizes nutritional benefits.

Cooking for specific dietary needs often requires careful consideration of ingredients and their health implications. Probiotics can be particularly beneficial for individuals with lactose intolerance, as fermented dairy products like yogurt and kefir contain lower levels of lactose compared to their non-fermented counterparts. Additionally, those following gluten-free diets can enjoy a variety of gluten-free fermented foods that are rich in probiotics, ensuring they do not miss out on the gut health benefits that fermentation offers. By highlighting these options, food lovers can create meals that are both satisfying and health-conscious. In conclusion, integrating probiotics into one's diet through fermented foods not only supports gut health but also enhances the overall culinary experience. The interplay between flavor, nutrition, and well-being opens up a world of possibilities for food lovers, encouraging exploration and creativity in the kitchen. By understanding the role of probiotics and their benefits, individuals can make informed choices that delight their palates while nurturing their digestive systems.

This approach not only celebrates the art of cooking but also empowers individuals to take charge of their health through the power of fermented delights.

Fermentation: A Historical Perspective
Fermentation has been an essential process in food preservation and flavor enhancement for thousands of years. Historical evidence suggests that the practice of fermenting foods dates back to ancient civilizations, with records indicating its use in Mesopotamia around 6000 BCE. This early form of food preservation allowed communities to store surplus crops and reduce waste, leading to a more stable food supply. Fermented products like bread, beer, and yogurt not only provided sustenance but also became integral to cultural practices, rituals, and social gatherings. As fermentation spread across different regions, it adapted to local ingredients and climate conditions, resulting in a diverse array of fermented foods that reflect regional culinary traditions.

In Asia, for instance, the fermentation of soybeans led to the creation of miso and soy sauce, while in Europe, the fermentation of milk gave rise to cheese and various yogurts. Each culture harnessed the power of fermentation not just for preservation but also for the unique flavors and textures that these processes imparted to the food. The art of fermentation thus became a cornerstone of culinary identity, showcasing the ingenuity of communities in utilizing natural processes to enhance their diet.

The health benefits of fermented foods have been recognized for centuries, often intertwined with cultural beliefs about wellness. Ancient societies were aware of the positive effects of these foods on digestion and overall health. For example, in traditional Chinese medicine, fermented foods were considered essential for maintaining balance within the body, promoting gut health and aiding digestion. By the 19th century, scientific advancements began to uncover the microbiological processes involved in fermentation, leading to a greater understanding of probiotics and their role in gut health. This combination of tradition and science has revitalized interest in fermented foods in modern diets. The 20th century saw a decline in home fermentation practices, largely due to the rise of industrial food production, which offered convenience but often sacrificed nutritional value. However, the resurgence of interest in artisanal and homemade foods has reignited the fermentation movement. Food lovers are increasingly turning to fermentation as a means to create flavorful, nutritious dishes while also catering to specific dietary needs.

The ability to customize fermented products allows for exploration in flavor pairing, where the synergistic effects of fermented foods can enhance the overall nutritional profile of meals.

Today, the historical journey of fermentation is not just a testament to its role in food preservation; it is a celebration of its potential to improve gut health and elevate culinary experiences. As food lovers embrace this ancient art, they are discovering the benefits of incorporating fermented foods into their diets, whether for enhancing flavors, improving digestion, or adapting to dietary restrictions. The legacy of fermentation continues to evolve, offering endless possibilities for creativity and wellness in the kitchen.

Chapter 2: The Gut Microbiome What is the Gut Microbiome? The gut microbiome refers to the diverse community of microorganisms residing in the human digestive tract, primarily in the intestines. This complex ecosystem consists of trillions of bacteria, viruses, fungi, and other microbes that play a crucial role in maintaining overall health. The composition of these microorganisms can vary greatly from person to person, influenced by factors such as diet, environment, age, and genetics.

Understanding the gut microbiome is vital for food lovers, especially those interested in fermentation and gut health, as it underscores the importance of dietary choices in shaping this microbial landscape. These microorganisms are not merely passive inhabitants; they actively participate in various physiological processes. They aid in the digestion of food, breaking down complex carbohydrates and fibers that the human body cannot digest on its own. This fermentation process produces short-chain fatty acids, which are essential for gut health and provide energy to nearby cells. Moreover, the gut microbiome plays a significant role in synthesizing certain vitamins, such as B vitamins and vitamin K, enhancing the nutritional value for those who enjoy cooking and eating nutrient-rich foods.

The balance of the gut microbiome is crucial for optimal health. A diverse and balanced microbiome is associated with a robust immune system, healthy metabolism, and even mental well-being. Conversely, an imbalance, often referred to as dysbiosis, can lead to various health issues, including digestive disorders, obesity, and autoimmune diseases. For food lovers interested in fermentation, fostering a healthy gut microbiome can be achieved through the incorporation of fermented foods, which are rich in probiotics—beneficial bacteria that can help restore balance. Fermented foods like yogurt, kefir, sauerkraut, and kimchi are not only delicious but also provide a multitude of health benefits. They are packed with live cultures that can enhance the diversity of the gut microbiome. By regularly consuming these foods, individuals can support their digestive health, improve nutrient absorption, and potentially reduce the risk of chronic diseases. For those focused on food pairing for enhanced nutrition, combining fermented foods with prebiotic-rich ingredients like garlic, onions, and whole grains can further nourish the gut microbiome, creating a symbiotic effect that boosts overall health.

Cooking for specific dietary needs can also benefit from a keen understanding of the gut microbiome. Personalized nutrition that takes into account individual microbiome profiles can lead to more effective dietary interventions. By tailoring meals to include both fermented foods and other gut-friendly ingredients, food lovers can create dishes that not only satisfy the palate but also promote gut health. This approach emphasizes the connection between flavor and health, allowing culinary enthusiasts to explore new tastes while nurturing their microbiome for a happier, healthier life. How Fermented Foods Influence the Microbiome

Fermented foods have gained significant attention in recent years, particularly for their profound influence on gut health and the microbiome. The microbiome consists of trillions of microorganisms living in our digestive tract, playing a crucial role in digestion, immune function, and overall health. Fermented foods, rich in probiotics, provide these beneficial bacteria essential for maintaining a balanced microbiome. The process of fermentation not only enhances the flavor of food but also increases its nutritional value, making it an appealing choice for food lovers who prioritize health. When we consume fermented foods, we introduce live microorganisms into our digestive system. These probiotics help populate the gut with beneficial bacteria, promoting a diverse microbiome. A diverse microbiome is linked to improved digestion and a reduced risk of various health issues, including gastrointestinal disorders, obesity, and even mood-related conditions. Popular fermented foods such as yogurt, kefir, sauerkraut, and kimchi are excellent sources of these probiotics, making them tasty additions to meals that support gut health.

Moreover, fermentation breaks down complex carbohydrates and proteins, making nutrients more bioavailable. This process can enhance the absorption of vitamins and minerals, particularly in foods that are traditionally hard to digest. For instance, the fermentation of grains can help reduce antinutrients like phytates, allowing for better mineral absorption. Food lovers can experiment with pairing fermented foods with other ingredients to create dishes that maximize nutritional benefits while also tantalizing the palate.

Fermented foods can be particularly beneficial for individuals with specific dietary needs. For example, those who are lactose intolerant may find that fermented dairy products like yogurt are easier to digest due to the presence of live cultures that help break down lactose. Similarly, individuals following gluten-free diets can enjoy fermented options made from gluten-free grains, which offer both flavor and probiotics. By understanding how to incorporate fermented foods into various dietary lifestyles, food enthusiasts can cater to their own health requirements while indulging in delightful flavors. Finally, the influence of fermented foods on the microbiome extends beyond individual health benefits; it also fosters a greater appreciation for traditional culinary practices and food cultures around the world. Fermentation has been used for centuries across various societies, each developing unique techniques and flavors that celebrate local ingredients. By embracing the art of fermentation, food lovers can not only enhance their meals but also connect with global traditions, enriching their culinary experiences while promoting gut health with every delicious bite.

Balancing Your Gut Health Balancing your gut health is essential for overall well-being, and fermentation plays a significant role in achieving this harmony. The gut is home to trillions of microorganisms, known as the gut microbiota, which contribute to digestion, nutrient absorption, and immune function. Incorporating fermented foods into your diet can help cultivate a diverse and balanced microbiota. Options such as yogurt, kefir, sauerkraut, and kimchi are rich in probiotics, which are beneficial bacteria that can enhance gut health by promoting a healthy balance of microorganisms. In addition to consuming probiotics, prebiotics are equally important for gut health. Prebiotics are non-digestible fibers found in certain foods that serve as food for probiotics. Foods such as garlic, onions, bananas, and asparagus are excellent sources of prebiotics.

By pairing fermented foods with prebiotic-rich ingredients, food lovers can create dishes that not only tantalize the taste buds but also support gut health. For instance, a yogurt-based dressing with garlic and herbs can be a delicious way to incorporate both probiotics and prebiotics into a meal. Cooking for specific dietary needs can also benefit from a focus on gut health. For individuals with lactose intolerance, using fermented dairy products like aged cheeses or lactose-free yogurt can provide the creamy texture and flavors they crave without the discomfort. Additionally, those following gluten-free diets can explore fermented options such as gluten-free sourdough bread. This not only enhances flavor but also improves digestibility, making it easier for individuals with sensitivities to enjoy baked goods without adverse effects. Food pairing is a crucial aspect of enhancing nutrition and flavor while supporting gut health.

Combining different fermented foods can create complex flavors while maximizing the health benefits. For example, pairing kimchi with grilled fish not only adds a spicy kick but also provides a rich source of omega-3 fatty acids, which are known to reduce inflammation and support gut health. Similarly, a salad featuring sauerkraut and avocado can offer a delightful combination of probiotics and healthy fats, making it a nutritious addition to any meal.

Ultimately, balancing your gut health through flavor involves being mindful of the foods you choose and how they complement one another. By focusing on a diverse range of fermented foods, incorporating prebiotics, and exploring creative food pairings, food lovers can enhance their culinary experiences while supporting their gut health. This holistic approach not only leads to improved digestion and overall wellness but also makes each meal an opportunity to celebrate the delightful flavors of fermented foods.

Chapter 3: Fermented Foods Around the World Kimchi: The Korean Superfood Kimchi, a staple of Korean cuisine, is increasingly recognized as a superfood, not just for its vibrant flavors but also for its profound health benefits. This fermented dish, primarily made from napa cabbage and Korean radishes, is typically seasoned with a blend of spices, garlic, ginger, and fish sauce. The fermentation process, often achieved through the natural action of lactic acid bacteria, not only preserves the vegetables but also enhances their nutritional profile.

As food lovers explore the realms of fermentation and gut health, kimchi stands out as an exemplary model of how traditional practices can yield foods that nourish both the body and the palate. The health benefits of kimchi are extensive, primarily attributed to its probiotic content. Probiotics, the beneficial bacteria that thrive in fermented foods, play a crucial role in gut health by promoting a balanced microbiome. A well-functioning gut microbiome is essential for proper digestion, nutrient absorption, and even immune function. Regular consumption of kimchi can support digestive health, alleviate conditions like irritable bowel syndrome, and reduce inflammation. For those keen on enhancing their gut health through flavorful foods, kimchi offers a delicious way to incorporate probiotics into their diet. In addition to its probiotic properties, kimchi is rich in vitamins and minerals, making it an excellent addition to any meal. The fermentation process increases the bioavailability of certain nutrients, allowing the body to absorb them more efficiently. Kimchi is particularly high in vitamins A, B, and C, as well as antioxidants that help combat oxidative stress.

For food lovers interested in pairing kimchi with other dishes, its bold flavors and crunchy texture can elevate everything from rice bowls to tacos, providing a nutritious boost while enhancing overall meal enjoyment.

For those with specific dietary needs, kimchi can be easily adapted to fit various lifestyles. Vegan and vegetarian versions exclude fish sauce, relying on plant-based ingredients for flavor, while gluten-free versions can be made without soy products. Additionally, the versatility of kimchi allows it to be incorporated into a range of culinary applications. Whether served as a side dish, used as a topping, or incorporated into stews and stir-fries, kimchi can complement many dietary preferences without sacrificing taste or nutrition. In conclusion, kimchi exemplifies how a traditional fermented food can serve as a modern superfood. Its rich flavors, coupled with numerous health benefits, make it a must-try for food lovers who appreciate the intersection of taste and nutrition. As interest in fermentation and gut health continues to grow, embracing kimchi not only enriches the dining experience but also contributes to a healthier lifestyle. By exploring the diverse ways to enjoy kimchi, enthusiasts can unlock its full potential, making it a delightful staple in their culinary repertoire.

Sauerkraut: A German Classic Sauerkraut, a staple of German cuisine, is a remarkable example of how fermentation not only enhances flavor but also contributes to gut health. Made from finely shredded cabbage that undergoes lactic acid fermentation, sauerkraut is rich in probiotics, vitamins, and minerals. This traditional preparation method dates back centuries, with origins tracing to ancient China and spreading through Europe, particularly Germany. The process involves simply mixing shredded cabbage with salt, which draws out moisture and creates an environment conducive to the growth of beneficial bacteria while inhibiting harmful pathogens. The health benefits of sauerkraut are significant, as it is loaded with probiotics that promote a healthy gut microbiome. These live microorganisms can improve digestion, boost the immune system, and even enhance mood regulation.

The fermentation process increases the availability of certain nutrients, such as vitamins C and K, and makes minerals like calcium and magnesium more bioavailable. For those focused on gut health, incorporating sauerkraut into meals can be a delicious way to support digestive wellness while exploring the rich flavors of this classic dish. When it comes to food pairing, sauerkraut is remarkably versatile. Its tangy, slightly sour flavor can complement a wide variety of dishes. Traditionally served alongside rich meats like sausages or roasted pork, the acidity of sauerkraut cuts through the fat, balancing the meal and enhancing the overall taste experience. It can also be used as a topping for sandwiches, adding crunch and a burst of flavor, or incorporated into salads and grain bowls to provide an extra layer of texture and nutrition.

For those with specific dietary needs, sauerkraut can be a gluten-free condiment that adds depth to a plethora of culinary creations.

For individuals following plant-based or low-carb diets, sauerkraut offers a nutritious option that aligns with their lifestyle choices. It can be enjoyed as a stand-alone side dish or as a flavorful addition to stir-fries and vegetable medleys. Incorporating sauerkraut into meals not only boosts the nutritional profile but also introduces a complex flavor that can elevate simple ingredients. Furthermore, the low-calorie nature of sauerkraut makes it a guilt-free indulgence, perfect for those who are mindful of their dietary intake. In conclusion, sauerkraut stands as a testament to the art of fermentation, marrying taste with nutrition in a way that appeals to food lovers across various dietary spectrums. Its rich history and numerous health benefits underscore the importance of this German classic in modern kitchens. Whether enjoyed as a side, a topping, or an ingredient, sauerkraut invites exploration and creativity, making it a delightful addition to any meal while promoting gut health and overall well-being.

Kefir and Yogurt: Dairy Delights Kefir and yogurt are two of the most celebrated dairy products in the realm of fermentation, both offering unique flavors and health benefits that make them staples in many diets. Originating from different cultural backgrounds, kefir hails from the Caucasus region, while yogurt has roots in various ancient civilizations across the globe. Both products are created through the fermentation of milk, but the distinct cultures used in their production result in varied textures, tastes, and nutritional profiles. This diversity not only enhances their appeal to food lovers but also provides numerous options for those seeking to improve their gut health. The fermentation process for both kefir and yogurt involves the action of beneficial bacteria and, in the case of kefir, yeast. Yogurt typically contains specific strains of bacteria such as Lactobacillus bulgaricus and Streptococcus thermophilus, leading to its creamy texture and mildly tangy flavor. On the other hand, kefir is made using kefir grains, a symbiotic culture of bacteria and yeasts, which produces a thicker, effervescent beverage that can be slightly tangy and sour.

The probiotic content in both products plays a significant role in supporting gut health by promoting a balanced microbiome, aiding digestion, and enhancing the immune system. In terms of nutritional value, both kefir and yogurt are excellent sources of protein, calcium, and B vitamins. However, kefir generally contains a higher concentration of probiotics, making it a more potent option for those looking to boost their gut health. Additionally, the fermentation process makes the nutrients in both products more bioavailable, allowing for improved absorption by the body. This quality makes them ideal candidates for food pairing, as they can complement a range of dishes while enhancing nutritional profiles. Pairing yogurt with fruits, nuts, or honey can create a delightful breakfast, while kefir can be utilized in smoothies, salad dressings, or even as a marinade for meats.

For individuals with specific dietary needs, both kefir and yogurt offer versatile options. Lactose-intolerant individuals may find kefir easier to digest due to its lower lactose content, resulting from the fermentation process in which lactose is broken down. Additionally, there are plant-based alternatives available, such as coconut or almond-based yogurts, that cater to vegan and dairy-free diets while still providing probiotic benefits. These alternatives allow food lovers to explore the world of fermented dairy delights without sacrificing taste or nutrition. Incorporating kefir and yogurt into daily meals not only enhances flavors but also supports overall health. From breakfast parfaits to savory dishes, the possibilities are endless. Experimenting with different flavor profiles—such as adding spices, herbs, or fruit—can elevate the culinary experience while promoting gut health. As food lovers continue to explore the myriad benefits of fermentation, kefir and yogurt stand out as delicious and nutritious options that can be enjoyed in a variety of ways. Miso and tempeh are two cornerstone ingredients in Japanese cuisine, celebrated not only for their rich flavors but also for their impressive health benefits.

Both products are derived from soybeans, yet they undergo distinct fermentation processes that impart unique nutritional profiles. Miso is a paste made by fermenting soybeans with salt and a specific mold called koji, while tempeh is created by fermenting cooked soybeans with a different mold, Rhizopus oligosporus. This divergence in fermentation not only enhances their taste but also affects their digestibility and nutritional content, making them essential staples for food lovers seeking to incorporate gut-healthy ingredients into their diets.

Miso is often lauded for its umami flavor, which can elevate a variety of dishes. It can be used in soups, dressings, marinades, and even desserts, showcasing its versatility. The fermentation process enriches miso with probiotics, which are beneficial for gut health. Additionally, miso is a source of protein, vitamins, and minerals, making it a valuable ingredient for those following vegetarian or vegan diets. Its salty, savory flavor can enhance the taste of vegetables and grains, providing a delicious way to boost nutritional value without relying on unhealthy additives. Tempeh, on the other hand, offers a firmer texture and a nutty flavor, making it an excellent meat substitute. The fermentation process converts the soybeans into a whole food that is easier to digest, allowing the body to absorb nutrients more effectively. Tempeh is rich in protein, fiber, and a range of essential nutrients, including iron and calcium. Its ability to absorb flavors makes it a perfect candidate for marinating and grilling, creating a satisfying and nutritious dish that caters to various dietary needs.

For those exploring food pairing, tempeh can complement grains and vegetables beautifully, enhancing both flavor and nutritional content. The combination of miso and tempeh in meals not only boosts flavor but also contributes to a balanced diet. When used together, they create a synergy that enhances the bioavailability of nutrients. For instance, pairing tempeh with a miso-based sauce can amplify the dish's protein content while introducing beneficial probiotics. This fusion is particularly appealing for food lovers interested in exploring culinary creativity while adhering to dietary restrictions or preferences. The balance of flavors and textures from both ingredients opens up a world of possibilities for health-conscious cooking.

Incorporating miso and tempeh into your culinary repertoire is an excellent way to celebrate the art of fermentation while prioritizing gut health. By experimenting with these Japanese staples, food lovers can create delicious and nutritious meals that cater to specific dietary needs. Whether it's a hearty miso soup, a grilled tempeh sandwich, or a flavorful stir-fry, the potential for innovative combinations is limitless. Embracing miso and tempeh not only enhances your cooking but also supports a thriving gut microbiome, ultimately leading to improved overall health and well-being. Fermented Beverages: Kombucha and Beyond Fermented beverages have surged in popularity in recent years, with kombucha often leading the charge. This effervescent drink, made from sweetened tea and a symbiotic culture of bacteria and yeast (SCOBY), offers a refreshing and tangy flavor profile that captivates the palate. Beyond its delightful taste, kombucha is lauded for its potential health benefits, particularly in promoting gut health.

Its natural carbonation and probiotics can aid digestion, improve gut flora balance, and possibly enhance overall wellness, making it a favored choice among food lovers who appreciate both flavor and nutrition. While kombucha remains a staple in the world of fermented drinks, there is a burgeoning array of other fermented beverages worth exploring. Kefir, for instance, is a tangy, yogurt-like drink made from fermented milk or water. It is rich in probiotics and can be easily incorporated into smoothies or enjoyed on its own. Similarly, kvass, a traditional Eastern European beverage made from fermented rye bread, offers a unique, slightly sour taste that pairs well with savory dishes. Each of these drinks provides distinct flavors and health benefits, catering to diverse palates and dietary preferences.

For food lovers interested in enhancing their culinary experiences, pairing fermented beverages with food can elevate meals to new heights. Kombucha's fruity and tart notes complement a variety of dishes, from spicy Asian cuisine to rich charcuterie boards. Kefir can add a creamy texture to salads and dressings or serve as a tangy counterpart to grilled meats. Kvass, with its earthy undertones, works beautifully with hearty stews and roasted vegetables. The interplay between the flavors of fermented drinks and dishes can enhance the overall dining experience while contributing to nutritional balance. Cooking for specific dietary needs can also be enriched through the inclusion of fermented beverages. For those on dairy-free diets, water kefir offers a probiotic-rich alternative that can be enjoyed without the lactose found in traditional dairy products. Gluten-free individuals can savor kvass made from gluten-free grains or fruits, allowing them to enjoy the benefits of fermentation without compromising their dietary restrictions. These beverages not only serve as functional ingredients but also as flavorful additions that can transform meals while supporting gut health.

Incorporating fermented beverages into daily routines is not just a trend; it is a lifestyle choice that embraces the richness of flavors and the benefits of fermentation. Experimenting with these drinks can inspire creativity in the kitchen, encouraging food lovers to explore new pairings and recipes. As we delve deeper into the world of fermented delights, we discover that the journey toward enhancing gut health can be both delicious and fulfilling, making each sip a testament to the power of fermentation in our diets.

Chapter 4: Getting Started with Home Fermentation

Tools and Equipment You'll Need

When embarking on your fermentation journey, having the right tools and equipment is essential for achieving optimal results. A few key items will make the process more efficient and enjoyable, ensuring that your fermented creations are both flavorful and beneficial for gut health. Start with a set of high-quality glass jars, preferably with wide mouths, as these allow for easy access during the fermentation process. Glass is non-reactive, which means it won't interfere with the flavors or health benefits of your ferment. Additionally, consider investing in fermentation weights to keep your ingredients submerged in their brine, preventing mold growth and ensuring a consistent fermentation environment. A good-quality food processor or blender is invaluable for preparing your ingredients. Chopping vegetables or blending fruits into a smooth puree can significantly enhance the fermentation process, allowing for better flavor integration and texture. For specific dietary needs, such as gluten-free or low-FODMAP diets, these tools can help you create tailored recipes that cater to your health goals.

A mandolin slicer can also be a great addition, especially for achieving uniform cuts that promote even fermentation in items like sauerkraut or pickles.

Temperature control is crucial in fermentation, as it can greatly influence the final taste and texture of your product. A reliable thermometer can help you monitor the temperature of your fermentation environment, ensuring that it remains within the ideal range for the specific type of fermentation you are undertaking. For those who wish to experiment with various fermentation styles, a dedicated fermentation crock can offer excellent temperature regulation. These crocks often come with water-sealed lids that create an anaerobic environment, essential for many fermented foods. Another important tool is a pH meter, which allows you to measure the acidity of your ferment. This is particularly useful for food lovers interested in the science of fermentation and its impact on gut health. Maintaining the right pH level can prevent spoilage and promote the growth of beneficial bacteria. Understanding the acidity of your ferments can also help with food pairing, as certain levels of acidity can complement specific flavors, enhancing both nutrition and enjoyment. Finally, don't overlook the importance of proper storage containers.

Once your fermentation is complete, transferring your products to airtight containers ensures freshness and longevity. Vacuum-seal bags or airtight glass containers can keep your ferments safe from spoilage while preserving their nutritional benefits. By equipping yourself with these essential tools and equipment, you will be well-prepared to create delicious and health-promoting fermented foods that not only please your palate but also support your overall well-being.

Basic Fermentation Techniques

Basic fermentation techniques are essential for anyone interested in enhancing their culinary repertoire while promoting gut health. Fermentation is a natural process that transforms food through the action of microorganisms such as bacteria, yeasts, and molds. This age-old technique not only preserves food but also enhances its flavor and nutritional profile. Understanding the fundamental methods of fermentation can empower food lovers to create their own vibrant, probiotic-rich foods at home. One of the simplest and most accessible fermentation techniques is lactic acid fermentation. This process occurs when sugars in food are converted into lactic acid by beneficial bacteria. Common examples include sauerkraut and kimchi, both made from cabbage. To initiate lactic fermentation, finely chop or shred the vegetables and mix them with salt. The salt draws out moisture, creating a brine in which the beneficial bacteria thrive. The mixture should be packed tightly into a jar and left at room temperature for several days to weeks, depending on the desired flavor and tanginess. This method not only preserves the vegetables but also enhances their digestibility and nutrient availability.

Another popular technique is alcoholic fermentation, primarily associated with beverages like beer and wine. In this process, yeast converts sugars into alcohol and carbon dioxide. Homebrewing can be an exciting venture for food enthusiasts looking to explore fermentation. To create a basic alcoholic beverage, one can start with a sugar source such as fruit or grains and add yeast. The mixture is then left to ferment in a controlled environment, allowing the yeast to work its magic. This technique not only results in delicious drinks but also introduces beneficial compounds that can support gut health when consumed in moderation.

Fermented dairy products, such as yogurt and kefir, represent another fascinating area of fermentation. These products are made by introducing specific strains of bacteria and sometimes yeast into milk. The fermentation process thickens the milk and results in a tangy flavor profile. To make yogurt at home, simply heat milk, cool it to a lukewarm temperature, and mix in a small amount of store-bought yogurt that contains live cultures. Allow the mixture to ferment in a warm place for several hours. This technique not only provides a probiotic-rich food but also offers versatility in cooking, as yogurt can be used in dressings, dips, and marinades.

Finally, it's important to consider the role of fermentation in enhancing food pairings for specific dietary needs. Fermented foods can complement a variety of ingredients, boosting their nutritional benefits and flavor profiles. For instance, pairing fermented vegetables with lean proteins or whole grains can create a balanced meal that supports gut health. Additionally, individuals following specific dietary plans, such as gluten-free or vegan diets, can benefit from incorporating fermented foods like miso, tempeh, or coconut yogurt, which provide essential nutrients while catering to their needs. By mastering basic fermentation techniques, food lovers can not only diversify their meals but also enhance their overall health and enjoyment of food.

Common Mistakes to Avoid

When venturing into the world of fermentation, food lovers often overlook some common pitfalls that can hinder their success and enjoyment. One major mistake is neglecting the importance of cleanliness. The fermentation process thrives on the balance of good bacteria, and any introduction of unwanted contaminants can spoil the batch. It is essential to sanitize all equipment thoroughly, including jars, utensils, and surfaces. This precaution not only protects your ferment but also ensures that you are cultivating a healthy environment for beneficial microbes to flourish. Another frequent error is not paying attention to the temperature at which fermentation occurs. Each type of ferment has its ideal temperature range, which significantly impacts the end product's flavor and texture. For example, lacto-fermented vegetables typically perform best at cooler temperatures, while dairy ferments like yogurt require a warmer environment. Ignoring these temperature guidelines can lead to underdeveloped flavors or even spoilage. Therefore, investing in a thermometer and understanding the specific needs of your ferments can elevate your culinary creations.

Time management is also crucial in the fermentation process. Many food lovers mistakenly rush the fermentation period, eager to taste their creations. However, each ferment has a specific time frame needed for development, and cutting this short can result in a bland or off-flavored product. It is essential to taste your ferments periodically, but resist the urge to consume them before they have reached their peak flavor. Patience is a virtue in fermentation, and allowing the process to unfold naturally will yield far more rewarding results.

Furthermore, many enthusiasts fail to consider the synergy of flavors when pairing fermented foods with other ingredients. Fermented products can have strong flavors that may overwhelm or clash with certain dishes. A common mistake is assuming that all fermented items complement each other equally. Instead, understanding the flavor profiles and nutritional benefits of various ferments can enhance your meals dramatically. Experimenting with different pairings can lead to delightful discoveries, but it is essential to approach this with a mindful consideration of balance and contrast.

Lastly, a significant misstep is not documenting your fermentation journey. Without keeping a journal of your processes, including ingredients, timings, and tasting notes, it becomes challenging to replicate successful batches or learn from past mistakes. This documentation serves as a valuable resource for future ferments, helping you refine your techniques and explore new possibilities. By avoiding these common mistakes, food lovers can fully embrace the joys of fermentation, enhancing both their culinary skills and gut health in the process.

Chapter 5: Flavor Profiles in Fermentation

Understanding Taste and Aroma

Taste and aroma play a crucial role in our overall eating experience, particularly in the realm of fermentation. The sensory interplay between these two elements not only enhances our enjoyment of food but also influences our health. Taste is primarily perceived through our taste buds, which detect five basic flavors: sweet, sour, salty, bitter, and umami. Each of these flavors can be amplified or altered through the fermentation process, creating a complex profile that can elevate a simple dish into something extraordinary. For instance, the natural sugars in fruits can be transformed into tangy notes during the fermentation of products like kombucha, while the umami flavors in soy sauce deepen with time, showcasing the magic of taste evolution.

Aroma, often closely linked with taste, is detected through our olfactory senses and contributes significantly to how we perceive flavor. Fermented foods are known for their distinctive aromas, which arise from the myriad of volatile compounds produced during fermentation. These compounds can range from fruity esters to pungent sulfur compounds, each contributing unique characteristics to the food. For food lovers, understanding the role of aroma can enhance the enjoyment of not just fermented products but also the overall culinary experience. Pairing foods thoughtfully, considering both taste and aroma, can create a more satisfying meal that supports gut health and nutritional goals.

The process of fermentation also introduces beneficial probiotics, which can impact our taste preferences. Research indicates that a healthy gut microbiome can influence our cravings and even our enjoyment of certain flavors. For those interested in gut health, consuming a variety of fermented foods can help diversify the gut flora, which in turn may lead to a broader appreciation for different tastes and aromas. This relationship underscores the importance of incorporating fermented delights into our diets, not only for their health benefits but also for their ability to enhance our sensory experiences around food.

When it comes to food pairing, understanding the balance of taste and aroma can significantly enhance nutritional intake. Certain flavors complement one another, creating a harmonious dish that nourishes both the body and the palate. For example, the acidity of fermented vegetables, such as sauerkraut, pairs beautifully with fatty foods like sausages, providing a balance that aids digestion. Similarly, incorporating fermented dairy, like yogurt, into savory dishes can add a creamy texture while introducing beneficial bacteria. By strategically combining flavors and aromas, food lovers can craft meals that are both delightful and health-promoting, catering to specific dietary needs.

In conclusion, a deep understanding of taste and aroma is essential for anyone passionate about food, especially in the context of fermentation and gut health. By appreciating the intricate relationships between these sensory experiences, we can create meals that not only satisfy our cravings but also support our overall well-being. Embracing fermented foods in our diets offers an exciting opportunity to explore new flavors and aromas, while also nurturing our gut health. As we continue to experiment with food pairings and cooking methods, we unlock the potential for enhanced nutrition, leading to a more vibrant and flavorful culinary journey.

Pairing Ingredients for Optimal Flavor

Pairing ingredients for optimal flavor is an art that enhances the culinary experience while also promoting gut health. Understanding how different flavors interact can transform your dishes into not only tasty meals but also nutritional powerhouses. The process of fermentation adds a unique layer to this pairing, as it introduces new flavors and health benefits. Ingredients that undergo fermentation, like sauerkraut or kimchi, can be paired with a variety of foods to create complex flavor profiles that tantalize the taste buds and support digestive health. One effective approach to pairing ingredients is to consider the balance of flavors—sweet, salty, sour, bitter, and umami. Fermented foods often exhibit pronounced sourness due to the lactic acid produced during fermentation. Pairing these tangy elements with rich, fatty ingredients can create a harmonious balance. For example, the acidity of fermented pickles complements the richness of fatty fish like salmon, enhancing the dish's flavor while also providing a beneficial combination of omega-3 fatty acids and probiotics that support gut health. Additionally, incorporating herbs and spices can elevate the flavor profile of fermented dishes.

Fresh herbs such as dill, cilantro, or basil can add brightness and freshness, countering the sometimes overpowering tang of fermented foods. Spices like turmeric and cumin not only contribute warmth and depth but also offer health benefits, including anti-inflammatory properties. These pairings can be particularly beneficial for those with dietary restrictions, as they allow for the creation of flavorful, nutrient-dense meals without relying on heavy or unhealthy ingredients.

Texture also plays a crucial role in flavor pairing. Fermented foods tend to have a crunchy or tangy texture that can contrast beautifully with creamy or smooth elements. For instance, a dollop of creamy avocado or yogurt on a fermented vegetable salad can create an appealing mouthfeel and enhance the overall sensory experience. This combination not only makes the dish more satisfying but also introduces healthy fats and probiotics, further supporting digestive health.

In conclusion, the art of pairing ingredients for optimal flavor is essential for both culinary delight and gut health. By considering the balance of flavors, incorporating fresh herbs and spices, and paying attention to texture, food lovers can create dishes that are not only delicious but also nourishing. Embracing the principles of fermentation allows for a greater exploration of flavors and health benefits, making every meal a celebration of taste and wellness.

The Art of Balancing Salt and Sugar

The balance of salt and sugar in cooking is an essential aspect of flavor development that can profoundly impact both taste and health. In the realm of fermentation, this balance becomes even more critical as it influences the fermenting agents, the final flavor profile, and the gut health benefits derived from the process. Salt is a natural preservative that inhibits harmful bacteria while promoting the growth of beneficial lactobacilli. Sugar, on the other hand, serves as food for these bacteria, aiding fermentation. Understanding how to balance these ingredients allows food lovers to create dishes that are not only delicious but also nutritionally advantageous. When considering the relationship between salt and sugar, it is important to recognize how they can enhance each other. A small amount of sugar can round out the sharpness of salt, creating a more nuanced flavor profile. This interplay is particularly evident in fermented foods like kimchi and sauerkraut, where the natural sweetness of vegetables is complemented by salt, resulting in a complex taste that elevates the overall dish.

By mastering the art of balancing these two elements, chefs and home cooks alike can craft ferments that are rich in flavor and beneficial to gut health. Moreover, the type of salt and sugar used can significantly affect the outcome of a dish. Sea salt, for example, can offer a briny depth that table salt lacks, while unrefined sugars such as honey or maple syrup provide not only sweetness but also additional nutrients and unique flavors. The choice of these ingredients should be guided by the intended flavor profile and health benefits. For those with specific dietary needs, such as low-sodium or low-sugar diets, there are numerous alternatives available, including potassium-based salts or natural sweeteners like stevia, which can help achieve the desired balance without compromising health.

In fermentation, the timing and method of introducing salt and sugar also play a crucial role. Adding salt too early can inhibit fermentation, while adding sugar too late may not allow sufficient time for beneficial bacteria to thrive. A careful approach, such as incorporating salt at the beginning of the fermentation process and sugar gradually throughout, can optimize both flavor and health benefits. This method encourages a robust fermentation process, yielding a product that is not only flavorful but also rich in probiotics, which are essential for gut health.

Ultimately, the art of balancing salt and sugar is about more than just flavor; it is a pathway to enhancing nutrition and promoting well-being. Food lovers can experiment with different ratios and combinations to discover what works best for their palate and dietary preferences. By embracing this balance in their cooking, they unlock a world of fermented delights that not only satisfy the taste buds but also nourish the gut, creating a holistic approach to health and flavor.

Chapter 6: Cooking with Fermented Foods

Incorporating Fermented Ingredients into Everyday Meals

Incorporating fermented ingredients into everyday meals can elevate not only the flavor profile of your dishes but also their nutritional value. Fermented foods are rich in probiotics, which contribute to gut health by promoting a balanced microbiome. By integrating these ingredients into common recipes, you can enhance both taste and health benefits without making drastic changes to your cooking habits. Simple adjustments can make a significant difference, allowing you to enjoy the delicious complexity and health advantages that fermentation offers.

One of the easiest ways to incorporate fermented ingredients is by adding fermented vegetables, such as kimchi or sauerkraut, to salads, sandwiches, and grain bowls. These tangy additions provide a crunch that complements the other textures in your meal while delivering probiotics. For instance, a classic coleslaw can be transformed by swapping out mayonnaise for a mix of yogurt and finely chopped kimchi, resulting in a creamy, spicy side that supports digestive health. Similarly, topping your sandwiches with sauerkraut adds depth of flavor and a beneficial probiotic punch, making your lunch both tasty and gut-friendly.

Fermented dairy products, like yogurt and kefir, can also be seamlessly integrated into your cooking. They can serve as bases for dressings, dips, or marinades, enhancing flavor while adding a creamy texture. A yogurt-based tzatziki sauce, paired with grilled meats or vegetables, not only contributes probiotics but also complements the dish with refreshing notes. Furthermore, using kefir in smoothies or baked goods can boost the nutritional profile of your breakfast or snacks. The tanginess of these fermented dairy options elevates ordinary recipes to new heights, making them more enjoyable and nutritious.

When cooking grains and legumes, consider using miso or tempeh to enrich your meals. Miso can be added to soups, dressings, and marinades to impart umami flavor while introducing beneficial microbes. Tempeh, a fermented soybean product, works well in stir-fries, salads, or sandwiches, providing a hearty protein source along with its probiotic content. By integrating these fermented ingredients, you not only enhance the taste but also support your dietary needs, whether you are vegetarian, vegan, or simply looking for nutritious alternatives.

Finally, don't overlook the potential of fermented beverages to complement your meals. Kombucha, kefir, or even fermented fruit drinks can serve as refreshing accompaniments to your culinary creations. They offer a unique flavor experience while contributing to your overall gut health. Pairing a tangy kombucha with a rich meal can create a balanced dining experience, enhancing the flavors of both the food and the drink. By thoughtfully incorporating fermented ingredients into your everyday meals, you can enjoy a flavorful journey toward better health and wellness, all while satisfying your culinary passions.

Fermented Sauces and Condiments

Fermented sauces and condiments play a vital role in enhancing the flavor profile of dishes while also contributing to gut health. These products are created through the process of fermentation, where beneficial bacteria break down sugars and starches, resulting in the production of lactic acid and other compounds that not only preserve the food but also enhance its nutritional value. Common examples include soy sauce, kimchi, miso, and various hot sauces. Each of these fermented condiments offers a unique taste and health benefits that food lovers can explore and incorporate into their culinary repertoire.

One of the key benefits of incorporating fermented sauces into meals is their role in promoting gut health. Fermented foods are rich in probiotics, which are live microorganisms that contribute to a healthy gut microbiome. A balanced microbiome is essential for digestion, nutrient absorption, and even mental health. For example, miso, made from fermented soybeans, is not only a flavorful addition to soups and marinades but also a source of beneficial bacteria that can aid in digestion. By adding these fermented condiments to your diet, you can enhance your gut flora and overall well-being. In addition to their health benefits, fermented sauces are incredibly versatile in food pairing. They can elevate a simple dish to new heights, enhancing flavors and adding depth. For instance, a splash of soy sauce can deepen the umami flavor in stir-fries, while a drizzle of kimchi juice can brighten up salads and grain bowls. The complexity of flavors brought by fermentation means that even a small amount can transform a dish, making it an essential tool for any food lover looking to create memorable meals.

Understanding how to pair these sauces with different ingredients can lead to more nutritious and delicious outcomes. For those with specific dietary needs, fermented sauces can also provide alternatives to traditional condiments that may not fit within certain dietary restrictions. For example, coconut aminos serve as a soy sauce substitute for those avoiding soy or gluten while still offering a similar depth of flavor. Fermented hot sauces, made from various peppers and vinegar, can provide a spicy kick without added preservatives or artificial ingredients, making them suitable for those seeking cleaner options. By exploring these alternatives, individuals can enjoy the benefits of fermentation while adhering to their dietary preferences.

In conclusion, fermented sauces and condiments not only enhance the taste of food but also support gut health and cater to various dietary needs. Their unique flavors can transform ordinary meals into extraordinary experiences, while the probiotics they contain contribute to a healthier digestive system. As food lovers embark on their culinary journeys, embracing fermented sauces can unlock new dimensions of flavor and nutrition, making every meal a delightful exploration of taste and health.

Creative Fermented Food Recipes

Creative fermentation offers an exciting avenue for food lovers to explore unique flavors while enhancing gut health. These recipes not only introduce new taste profiles but also incorporate the beneficial bacteria that fermentation provides. The process of fermentation transforms ordinary ingredients into culinary delights, making them more digestible and nutritious. For those interested in gut health, these creative recipes will not only tantalize the palate but also support overall well-being. One delightful recipe to consider is a spicy kimchi made with seasonal vegetables like radishes, carrots, and napa cabbage. This traditional Korean staple is not just a side dish; it can be transformed into a vibrant topping for tacos or a zesty addition to grain bowls. The key to a successful kimchi is balancing the heat of gochugaru with the umami of fermented fish sauce or a vegan alternative like miso. These ingredients work together to create a depth of flavor that enhances the dish while promoting gut health through the probiotics produced during fermentation.

Another innovative recipe is the creation of fermented salsa, which combines the tang of tomatoes, the freshness of cilantro, and the zing of lime juice. This salsa can be left to ferment for several days, allowing the flavors to meld and develop a complexity that fresh salsa lacks. It can be paired with grilled meats, used as a dip for vegetables, or drizzled over roasted sweet potatoes. Not only does this fermented salsa add a burst of flavor, but it also provides beneficial bacteria that support digestive health.

For those cooking with specific dietary needs, consider a fermented nut cheese made from cashews or almonds. This dairy-free alternative can be seasoned with herbs and spices, providing a rich and creamy texture that works well on crackers or as a spread. The fermentation process not only enhances the flavor, making it tangy and satisfying, but also breaks down the nuts, making them easier to digest. This recipe is ideal for those avoiding dairy while still wanting to enjoy cheese-like flavors.

Finally, a refreshing fermented drink, such as ginger bug soda, can be a fun addition to any meal. By fermenting ginger, sugar, and water, you create a naturally fizzy beverage that can be flavored with fruits or herbs. This drink not only quenches thirst but also delivers probiotics that contribute to gut health. Pair it with spicy dishes or enjoy it as a standalone refreshment. These creative recipes showcase how fermentation can elevate everyday foods while promoting a healthy gut.

Chapter 7: Dietary Needs and Fermented Foods

Fermentation for Gut Health in Specific Diets

Fermentation is a centuries-old culinary process that not only enhances the flavor of foods but also plays a pivotal role in promoting gut health. For food lovers interested in the intricate relationship between diet and digestion, understanding how fermentation can benefit specific dietary needs is essential. Fermented foods, such as yogurt, kimchi, sauerkraut, and kombucha, are rich in probiotics, which are live microorganisms that contribute positively to gut flora. This diverse ecosystem of bacteria supports digestion, boosts the immune system, and can even influence mood and mental health.

In specific diets, such as vegetarian or vegan, fermented foods can serve as an excellent source of essential nutrients often lacking in plant-based diets. For instance, fermented soy products like tempeh not only provide protein but also enhance the bioavailability of vitamins and minerals. The fermentation process breaks down anti-nutrients found in raw legumes and grains, making essential nutrients more accessible. Additionally, incorporating fermented vegetables into meals can bolster fiber intake, promoting regularity and overall digestive health, which is particularly important for those adhering to plant-based diets.

For individuals following gluten-free diets, fermented foods are equally beneficial. Foods like gluten-free sourdough bread utilize fermentation to improve digestibility. The fermentation process helps to break down gluten proteins and enhances the absorption of nutrients, making the final product more gut-friendly. Fermented beverages like kefir can also be made using non-dairy milks, providing a creamy, probiotic-rich alternative for those avoiding gluten and dairy. Such adaptations not only maintain flavor and texture but also ensure that those with dietary restrictions can still enjoy the benefits of fermentation.

Food pairing is another crucial aspect of optimizing gut health through fermentation. Combining fermented foods with other nutrient-dense ingredients can enhance their health benefits. For example, pairing sauerkraut with lean meats or fish can aid in protein digestion, while serving yogurt with fiber-rich fruits can promote a balanced meal that supports gut health. Understanding these combinations can elevate the dining experience, allowing food lovers to enjoy both taste and nutrition. This mindful approach to food pairing ensures that each meal contributes positively to overall digestive health.

Finally, the benefits of fermentation extend beyond individual ingredients; they also enrich cultural and culinary traditions. Exploring global cuisines that emphasize fermented foods can inspire creativity in the kitchen. From Asian kimchi to European pickles, these diverse flavors can be integrated into various diets, bringing excitement and complexity to meals. By embracing fermentation, food lovers can not only enhance their culinary repertoire but also take meaningful steps toward improving their gut health, making every bite a delightful experience.

Vegan and Vegetarian Fermented Options

Vegan and vegetarian fermented options offer a wealth of flavors and health benefits, making them an excellent choice for food lovers seeking to enhance their diets. Fermentation is a process that not only preserves food but also enriches it with probiotics, which can improve gut health and boost overall wellness. For those following plant-based diets, the range of fermented foods available is extensive, providing both nutrition and culinary excitement. From tangy sauerkraut to creamy cashew yogurt, these options cater to diverse palates and dietary needs. One of the most popular fermented foods is sauerkraut, made from finely shredded cabbage that undergoes lactic acid fermentation. It is rich in vitamins C and K, as well as gut-friendly probiotics. Sauerkraut can be easily incorporated into meals, adding a zesty flavor to sandwiches, salads, or as a side dish. Additionally, kimchi, a Korean staple, offers a spicy alternative. Made from fermented vegetables, usually Napa cabbage and radishes, kimchi is packed with antioxidants and can provide a satisfying kick to rice bowls or tacos.

Fermented plant-based dairy alternatives also play a significant role in vegan and vegetarian diets. Coconut yogurt and almond-based yogurts are popular choices that retain the creamy texture of traditional dairy while providing beneficial bacteria. These products can be enjoyed on their own, blended into smoothies, or used as a base for salad dressings. The fermentation process not only enhances flavor but also increases the bioavailability of nutrients, making them easier for the body to absorb.

Another exciting option is miso, a fermented soybean paste that is a staple in Japanese cuisine. Miso is versatile and can be used to create soups, marinades, and dressings. It is packed with essential amino acids and probiotics, making it a nutritious addition to any meal. Pairing miso with seasonal vegetables in stir-fries or incorporating it into dipping sauces can elevate dishes while providing a depth of flavor that is both savory and satisfying.

Lastly, kombucha, a fermented tea, has gained popularity for its refreshing taste and probiotic content. This fizzy beverage can be found in various flavors, from classic ginger to fruity berry blends. Kombucha is not only a delightful drink but also an excellent way to support digestive health. Pairing it with a light meal, such as a salad or sushi, can create a harmonious dining experience that amplifies the health benefits of both food and drink. Embracing these vegan and vegetarian fermented options allows food lovers to explore new flavors while nurturing their gut health effectively.

Gluten-Free Fermentation Alternatives

Gluten-free fermentation alternatives offer an exciting avenue for food lovers seeking to explore the world of gut health while accommodating specific dietary needs. Traditional fermentation processes often rely on gluten-containing grains such as wheat, barley, and rye. However, a variety of gluten-free options can be utilized to create delicious, health-promoting fermented foods. These alternatives not only provide a safe option for those with gluten sensitivities but also introduce unique flavors and textures that can enhance culinary creativity.

One popular gluten-free fermentation option is using grains such as rice, millet, or quinoa. These grains can be transformed into a variety of fermented products, from tangy rice miso to light and airy quinoa sourdough. Each grain brings its distinct flavor profile and nutritional benefits to the table. For instance, quinoa is a complete protein, making it an excellent choice for those looking to boost their protein intake while enjoying fermented foods. By experimenting with different grains, food lovers can create a diverse array of fermented delights that cater to their taste preferences and dietary restrictions.

Legumes also present a remarkable alternative for fermentation, particularly for those avoiding gluten. Fermented bean pastes, such as tempeh and miso, provide rich umami flavors while offering a plethora of health benefits. Tempeh, made from fermented soybeans, is not only a source of protein but also contains prebiotics that promote a healthy gut microbiome. Additionally, chickpeas can be used to create fermented spreads like hummus, which can be enhanced with probiotics through the fermentation process. These legume-based options not only satisfy the palate but also contribute to overall gut health.

Fruits and vegetables are another exciting realm for gluten-free fermentation. From classic sauerkraut and kimchi to fruit-based ferments like kombucha and fruit kvass, the possibilities are endless. Fermenting vegetables enhances their nutritional profile by increasing the bioavailability of vitamins and minerals while introducing gut-friendly probiotics. On the other hand, fruit ferments can provide a delightful sweetness and complexity, making them perfect for pairing with a variety of dishes. Both categories offer a wealth of flavors that can complement meals and snacks, encouraging food lovers to embrace the vibrant world of fermented produce.

Incorporating gluten-free fermentation alternatives into daily meals not only caters to specific dietary needs but also enhances overall nutrition and flavor. By embracing diverse ingredients such as gluten-free grains, legumes, and produce, food enthusiasts can create a range of delicious and healthful options that support gut health. As the interest in fermentation continues to grow, the exploration of gluten-free alternatives not only expands culinary horizons but also fosters a deeper understanding of the relationship between food, flavor, and well-being.

Chapter 8: Pairing Fermented Foods with Other Ingredients

Enhancing Nutrition through Food Pairing

Enhancing nutrition through food pairing is a powerful strategy that not only elevates the flavor of meals but also maximizes their health benefits. By combining certain foods, we can create synergistic effects that improve nutrient absorption and enhance our overall well-being. This is particularly relevant for food lovers who are passionate about both taste and health, as well as those who explore the intricacies of fermentation and gut health. The process of pairing foods thoughtfully allows us to create dishes that are not only delicious but also nutritionally rich.

One of the most significant aspects of food pairing is the concept of complementary nutrients. For instance, pairing a vitamin C-rich food, such as bell peppers or citrus fruits, with iron-rich foods like leafy greens or legumes can greatly enhance iron absorption. This is particularly beneficial for individuals with specific dietary needs, such as vegetarians or those with anemia. By understanding how different nutrients interact, we can craft meals that support our body's requirements while still satisfying our taste buds.

Fermented foods play a crucial role in this nutritional enhancement. Probiotics found in fermented products like yogurt, kimchi, and sauerkraut can improve gut health, aiding in digestion and nutrient absorption. When combined with fiber-rich foods like whole grains or beans, the effects are compounded. The fermentation process itself breaks down complex carbohydrates, making the nutrients more accessible. Thus, food lovers can enjoy the rich flavors of fermented dishes while simultaneously boosting their nutritional profile through smart pairings.

Spices and herbs also contribute significantly to food pairing strategies. Not only do they enhance flavor, but many spices have anti-inflammatory and antioxidant properties that can further support gut health. For example, turmeric paired with black pepper enhances the bioavailability of curcumin, the active compound in turmeric, amplifying its health benefits. Incorporating these elements into meals can turn an ordinary dish into a powerhouse of nutrition, appealing to both the palate and the body's needs.

Ultimately, enhancing nutrition through food pairing is about creating a holistic approach to eating. By being mindful of how different foods interact, we can design meals that cater to our taste preferences while also meeting our health goals. This approach encourages a deeper appreciation for the culinary arts, inviting food lovers to explore new combinations and techniques that not only tantalize the senses but also contribute to a healthier lifestyle. Embracing the principles of food pairing enriches our culinary experiences and empowers us to make informed choices for our bodies and well-being.

Fermented Foods and Their Complementary Flavors

Fermented foods are a treasure trove of flavors, offering a diverse range of tastes and textures that can enhance any culinary experience. From tangy sauerkraut to creamy yogurt, these foods not only contribute to gut health but also serve as a foundation for exploring complementary flavors in cooking. Understanding how to pair fermented foods with various ingredients can elevate dishes, making them not only nutritious but also gastronomically exciting. By delving into the nuances of flavor profiles, food lovers can unlock the full potential of these fermented delights.

One of the most popular fermented foods, kimchi, exemplifies the art of flavor pairing. Its spicy, tangy, and umami-rich components can be beautifully complemented by milder flavors such as avocado or mango. Incorporating these fruits into a salad or a wrap can create a balanced dish that harmonizes the boldness of kimchi with creamy and sweet notes. Additionally, the crunch of fresh vegetables can add texture, enhancing the overall eating experience. This synergy between the sharpness of fermented foods and the subtler flavors of fresh produce can lead to satisfying meals that support gut health.

Yogurt, another staple in the world of fermentation, presents numerous opportunities for creative pairings. Its creamy texture and tartness make it a versatile ingredient in both savory and sweet dishes. For instance, combining yogurt with herbs like dill or mint can create a refreshing dip or dressing that complements grilled meats or roasted vegetables. On the sweeter side, pairing yogurt with honey and seasonal fruits can transform it into a delightful breakfast or dessert. These combinations not only enhance flavor but also contribute to a balanced intake of nutrients, catering to various dietary needs.

Miso, a fermented soybean paste, adds depth to dishes with its rich umami flavor. It pairs exceptionally well with ingredients like ginger, garlic, and scallions, making it a fantastic base for soups, marinades, and dressings. When combined with lighter proteins such as fish or chicken, miso can elevate the dish while providing a gut-friendly boost. Additionally, incorporating miso into salad dressings can enhance the flavor profile while ensuring that the meal remains nutritious. This versatility showcases how fermented foods can be seamlessly integrated into different cuisines, appealing to a wide range of palates.

Exploring the world of fermented foods also opens doors to unique flavor pairings that are not commonly considered. For example, the tangy notes of pickled vegetables can enhance the richness of fatty foods like cheese or oily fish. Pairing pickles with a charcuterie board can create a delightful contrast that excites the palate. Similarly, the acidity of fermented drinks, such as kombucha, can cut through the richness of creamy desserts, offering a refreshing finish to a meal. By embracing the complementary flavors of fermented foods, food lovers can create dishes that are not only beneficial for gut health but also satisfying and memorable.

Creating Balanced Meals with Fermented Ingredients

Creating balanced meals with fermented ingredients involves understanding how these foods can enhance both flavor and nutritional value. Fermentation not only preserves food but also transforms it into a source of probiotics, which play a vital role in gut health. This process increases the bioavailability of essential nutrients, making fermented foods a valuable addition to any meal. By incorporating these ingredients, food lovers can create dishes that are both satisfying and beneficial for their digestive systems.

When planning meals, consider the principles of food pairing to enhance the nutritional profile of your dishes. Fermented ingredients, such as kimchi, sauerkraut, yogurt, and miso, can be combined with various foods to create a harmonious balance. For instance, a vibrant salad incorporating fermented vegetables can be paired with whole grains, like quinoa or faro, to provide a complete amino acid profile. Adding a source of healthy fats, such as avocado or nuts, can further enhance the meal's satiety and nutrient absorption, making it a well-rounded option.

Incorporating fermented ingredients into specific dietary needs can be both innovative and delicious. For those following gluten-free diets, fermented grains like buckwheat or quinoa can be used as the base for bowls, topped with fermented sauces or pickled vegetables. Vegan diets can benefit from the umami flavor of fermented ingredients like nutritional yeast or miso, which can add depth to plant-based meals. Understanding how to utilize these ingredients allows for the creation of meals that cater to various dietary preferences without sacrificing taste or nutrition.

Texture is another important aspect to consider when creating balanced meals with fermented ingredients. The crunchiness of pickled vegetables can add an appealing contrast to creamy elements, such as avocado or tahini. Fermented dairy products, like kefir or yogurt, can provide a smooth and tangy component that complements richer foods. By thoughtfully combining different textures, food lovers can elevate their dining experience while ensuring their meals are nourishing and enjoyable.

Lastly, experimenting with fermented ingredients opens the door to endless culinary creativity. Embrace the versatility of fermentation by incorporating it into various cuisines. From a Korean-inspired bibimbap topped with gochujang and kimchi to a Mediterranean spread featuring tzatziki and olives, the possibilities are vast. Through this exploration, not only do you enhance your meals, but you also promote gut health, making every bite a flavorful step toward well-being.

Chapter 9: The Future of Fermentation

Innovations in Fermented Food Products

Innovations in fermented food products have surged in recent years, driven by a growing understanding of the health benefits associated with gut health. As consumers become more health-conscious, the demand for foods that support digestive wellness has led to an explosion of creativity in the fermentation space. New techniques and ingredients are emerging, which not only enhance the flavor profile of traditional fermented foods but also broaden their appeal to a wider audience. This evolution invites food lovers to explore a diverse array of options that cater to various dietary needs and preferences.

One notable innovation is the incorporation of non-traditional ingredients into the fermentation process. For instance, plant-based milks, such as oat, almond, and coconut, are being fermented to create dairy-free yogurts and cheeses. These products not only cater to lactose-intolerant individuals but also appeal to vegans and those seeking to reduce their dairy intake. By using live cultures, these alternative products can maintain the probiotic benefits associated with traditional dairy fermentations while offering unique flavors and textures that enhance culinary experiences.

In addition to ingredient innovation, the fermentation process itself has seen advancements. Techniques such as controlled fermentation and the use of specific bacterial strains allow producers to fine-tune the flavor, texture, and probiotic content of their products. For example, some companies are experimenting with rapid fermentation methods that significantly reduce the time required to produce fermented foods without sacrificing quality. This efficiency not only meets consumer demand for fresh products but also allows for greater accessibility of gut-friendly foods in the marketplace.

Food pairing has also evolved alongside these innovations, with an emphasis on enhancing nutritional value and flavor profiles. Chefs and food enthusiasts are discovering that pairing fermented foods with complementary ingredients can amplify both their health benefits and culinary appeal. For instance, combining fermented vegetables with high-fiber grains creates a balanced dish that supports digestive health while providing a satisfying meal. These innovative pairings encourage creativity in the kitchen and inspire home cooks to experiment with their own combinations, making fermentation a more integral part of everyday cooking.

As the landscape of fermented food products continues to evolve, it is clear that these innovations are not just trends but rather significant shifts in how we approach food and nutrition. The integration of novel ingredients, advanced fermentation techniques, and thoughtful food pairings all contribute to a richer, more diverse culinary experience. For food lovers passionate about fermentation and gut health, these innovations provide exciting opportunities to explore and enjoy the myriad flavors and benefits that fermented foods have to offer.

The Role of Fermentation in Sustainable Eating

Fermentation has emerged as a vital practice in the realm of sustainable eating, offering a multifaceted approach to food preservation, flavor enhancement, and nutritional enrichment. This ancient technique not only extends the shelf life of various foods but also enriches them with beneficial probiotics. These live microorganisms contribute significantly to gut health, promoting a balanced microbiome that is essential for overall well-being. As food lovers increasingly seek ways to enhance their diets sustainably, understanding the fermentation process can open doors to a world of flavors while simultaneously supporting health.

The fermentation process is driven by microorganisms such as bacteria, yeast, and molds, which break down sugars and starches in food, creating a variety of byproducts like lactic acid, ethanol, and carbon dioxide. These byproducts not only impart unique flavors but also create an environment that inhibits spoilage-causing pathogens. Fermented foods, including yogurt, kimchi, and sauerkraut, are prime examples of how this technique can transform simple ingredients into nutritional powerhouses. By incorporating these foods into our diets, we not only relish their complex tastes but also harness their health benefits, contributing to a more sustainable approach to eating.

In the context of food pairing, fermentation plays a crucial role in enhancing the nutritional profile of meals. Combining fermented foods with fresh ingredients can create a synergistic effect, elevating the overall nutrient absorption. For instance, pairing a tangy fermented salsa with grilled vegetables not only adds a burst of flavor but also boosts the bioavailability of vitamins and minerals. This mindful approach to food pairing can help individuals with specific dietary needs meet their nutritional requirements while enjoying a diverse and satisfying culinary experience.

Moreover, fermentation aligns with the principles of sustainable eating by promoting the use of local and seasonal ingredients. By fermenting surplus produce, individuals can reduce food waste and make the most of what is readily available. This practice supports local farmers and encourages a more environmentally conscious approach to meal preparation. The ability to transform excess fruits and vegetables into delicious fermented products empowers food lovers to explore creativity in the kitchen while contributing to a more resilient food system.

Embracing fermentation as part of a sustainable eating philosophy not only enhances culinary experiences but also fosters a deeper connection to food. By understanding the role of fermentation in gut health, nutrition, and sustainability, food enthusiasts can cultivate a more mindful approach to their diets. This not only enriches their palates but also supports a healthier planet, illustrating that the journey toward better eating is as much about flavor as it is about responsibility. As we unlock the delights of fermentation, we can savor the taste of sustainability in every bite.

Exploring New Trends in Gut Health

The field of gut health is evolving rapidly, with new trends emerging that highlight the importance of fermentation and its impact on the microbiome. As food lovers become increasingly aware of the profound connection between diet and health, fermentation has taken center stage. This ancient practice, which enhances flavor and preserves food, is now recognized for its ability to cultivate beneficial bacteria, improve digestion, and bolster the immune system. From kimchi to kombucha, fermented foods are not only delightful to the palate but also play a crucial role in maintaining a healthy gut.

Recent research underscores the significance of diversity in our diets, particularly when it comes to gut health. A varied intake of fruits, vegetables, and fermented products can promote a diverse microbiome, which is essential for optimal health. Trends indicate a growing interest in incorporating a wider array of fermented foods into daily meals. This shift is not just about adding probiotics; it's about enhancing the overall nutritional profile of dishes. By pairing fermented foods with fresh ingredients and whole grains, food lovers can create meals that are both delicious and nutritionally rich.

Food pairing strategies are also evolving, as enthusiasts discover how certain combinations can enhance the benefits of fermented foods. For instance, pairing yogurt with high-fiber fruits can improve digestion and nutrient absorption. Similarly, incorporating fermented sauces into dishes can elevate flavors while providing probiotics. This trend encourages culinary creativity, inviting home cooks to experiment with various ingredients that complement the health benefits of fermentation. By understanding which foods pair well, individuals can craft meals that support their dietary needs while tantalizing their taste buds.

Another significant trend is the customization of fermented foods to cater to specific dietary requirements. As awareness of food sensitivities and allergies increases, manufacturers and home cooks alike are creating innovative products that accommodate these needs. For example, dairy-free yogurts made from coconut or almond milk are gaining popularity among those with lactose intolerance. Additionally, gluten-free fermented breads and snacks are making it easier for individuals with celiac disease to enjoy the benefits of fermentation without compromising their health. This trend not only broadens accessibility but also encourages inclusivity in the culinary world.

As these trends in gut health continue to evolve, the intersection of flavor, nutrition, and fermentation offers exciting opportunities for food lovers. Embracing new practices and experimenting with diverse ingredients can lead to a deeper understanding of how food affects our well-being. By prioritizing gut health through flavorful, fermented options, individuals can enhance their overall dietary experience. The journey into the world of fermented delights is not just about savoring unique tastes; it's about unlocking the potential for better health, one delicious bite at a time.

Chapter 10: Conclusion: Embracing Fermented Delights

Building a Fermented Food Routine

Building a fermented food routine can transform not only your palate but also your gut health. Incorporating fermented foods into your daily diet is a flavorful way to enhance your nutrition and promote well-being. Start by understanding the types of fermented foods available, such as yogurt, kefir, sauerkraut, kimchi, and kombucha. Each offers unique flavors and health benefits, making them versatile additions to various meals. By familiarizing yourself with these options, you can better integrate them into your daily routine.

To establish a successful routine, begin with small changes. Aim to include one serving of fermented food in at least one meal each day. For instance, you might enjoy a bowl of yogurt topped with fresh fruit for breakfast or add a scoop of sauerkraut to a sandwich at lunch. As you become more comfortable, gradually increase the frequency and variety of fermented foods you consume. Experimentation is key; try different combinations and recipes to discover what excites your taste buds while reaping the health benefits of fermentation.

Pairing fermented foods with other nutrient-dense ingredients can enhance their health benefits. Consider how fermented foods can complement various dishes. For example, a tangy kimchi can elevate the flavor of a stir-fry or serve as a spicy topping for tacos. Yogurt can be used as a creamy base for salad dressings or smoothies, while fermented beverages like kombucha can be enjoyed alongside meals for a refreshing contrast. By thoughtfully incorporating these foods into your meals, you not only enhance your nutrient intake but also create a more balanced, satisfying eating experience.

For those with specific dietary needs, fermented foods can be tailored to suit individual preferences. Gluten-free grains can be used to create delicious gluten-free sourdough bread, while dairy-free options abound, such as almond or coconut yogurt. It's essential to consider the ingredients and methods used in fermentation to ensure they align with your dietary restrictions. This adaptability encourages everyone, regardless of dietary needs, to embrace the benefits of fermented foods while enjoying flavorful meals.

Finally, consistency is vital in building a fermented food routine. Keep your kitchen stocked with a variety of fermented foods to encourage daily consumption. Set reminders or create meal plans that feature these items, making it easier to incorporate them into your lifestyle. Over time, you will develop a habit that not only supports gut health but also enriches your culinary experiences. As you continue to explore and enjoy the world of fermentation, you'll find that these vibrant foods can play a central role in your journey toward enhanced nutrition and overall well-being.

The Journey to Better Gut Health

The journey to better gut health begins with understanding the crucial role our gut microbiome plays in overall well-being. This complex ecosystem of microorganisms influences digestion, immunity, and even mental health. For food lovers, this opens a world of opportunities to explore flavors and ingredients that not only tantalize the taste buds but also nourish our microbiomes. Embracing this journey means focusing on foods that promote the growth of beneficial bacteria, which can be achieved through the delicious practice of fermentation.

Fermented foods, such as yogurt, kimchi, sauerkraut, and kombucha, are rich in probiotics that enhance gut health. These live bacteria support digestion, help balance the gut flora, and can even alleviate symptoms of digestive disorders. Incorporating a variety of fermented delights into your diet can create a diverse microbiome, which is essential for optimal health. The process of fermentation itself adds unique flavors and textures to food, making it an exciting avenue for food lovers to explore new culinary experiences while reaping health benefits.

In addition to incorporating fermented foods, food pairing is a vital aspect of enhancing nutrition. Certain combinations can amplify the absorption of nutrients and foster a more favorable environment for gut health. For instance, pairing fiber-rich foods with fermented options can create a synergistic effect, promoting the growth of beneficial bacteria. Foods like whole grains, fruits, and vegetables provide prebiotics, the non-digestible fibers that feed probiotics. By thoughtfully combining these foods, one can create meals that are not only flavorful but also supportive of gut health.

Cooking for specific dietary needs does not have to mean sacrificing taste. In fact, many alternative diets can benefit significantly from the inclusion of fermented foods. For those following gluten-free, dairy-free, or vegan diets, there are numerous options for creating delicious fermented delights that cater to their needs. Exploring alternatives like coconut yogurt or fermented nut cheeses can introduce new flavors and textures to meals while supporting gut health. These adaptations encourage creativity and innovation in the kitchen, allowing food lovers to indulge in their passion without compromising their dietary restrictions.

Ultimately, the journey to better gut health is about discovering the intersection of flavor and nutrition. By embracing fermentation and understanding the importance of food pairing, anyone can enhance their culinary repertoire while nurturing their gut microbiome. This journey invites food lovers to experiment, learn, and share their experiences, creating a vibrant community that celebrates both delicious food and healthful living. As we unlock the potential of fermented delights, we can enjoy a richer, more flavorful life while supporting our health in the process.

Encouraging Exploration and Experimentation

Encouraging exploration and experimentation in the kitchen is essential for food lovers who wish to enhance their understanding of fermentation and gut health. The process of fermentation is not just about following a recipe; it is an invitation to engage with ingredients in a dynamic way. Each fermentation project offers unique flavors, textures, and nutritional benefits, encouraging individuals to step outside their comfort zones. By trying new fermentation techniques or using unconventional ingredients, home cooks can discover personal preferences and develop a deeper appreciation for the transformative power of fermentation.

Exploration in the realm of fermentation can be particularly rewarding when considering the myriad of food pairings that can enhance nutritional profiles. For instance, pairing fermented foods with fresh produce can amplify both flavor and health benefits. Experimenting with different combinations, such as kimchi with avocado or yogurt with leafy greens, not only creates exciting dishes but also promotes a more varied intake of nutrients. Encouraging this kind of culinary creativity allows individuals to find harmony in flavors while maximizing the benefits of both fermented and fresh ingredients.

For those with specific dietary needs or restrictions, encouraging exploration can lead to the development of personalized recipes that cater to individual health goals. Gluten-free grains, dairy alternatives, and low-sugar options can all be incorporated into fermentation practices, allowing individuals to enjoy the benefits of gut-friendly foods without compromising their dietary requirements. This adaptability fosters an environment where home cooks can tweak traditional recipes and innovate new ones, ensuring that everyone can partake in the delights of fermentation while adhering to their unique health needs.

Additionally, the act of experimentation can demystify the fermentation process, making it less intimidating for beginners. By trying small batches of different fermented foods, such as sauerkraut, kefir, or kombucha, individuals can learn through trial and error. Documenting results, whether successful or not, can provide valuable insights into flavor development and fermentation dynamics. This hands-on approach cultivates a sense of confidence and competence in the kitchen, encouraging people to take pride in their culinary endeavors while emphasizing the importance of patience and observation in the fermentation process.

Ultimately, fostering an environment that encourages exploration and experimentation not only enhances the enjoyment of food but also contributes to better health outcomes. The journey of discovering new flavors, understanding the science behind fermentation, and adapting recipes to fit specific dietary needs can transform how individuals view their relationship with food. By embracing this spirit of adventure, food lovers can unlock the full potential of fermented delights, enriching their diets and supporting their gut health in the process.

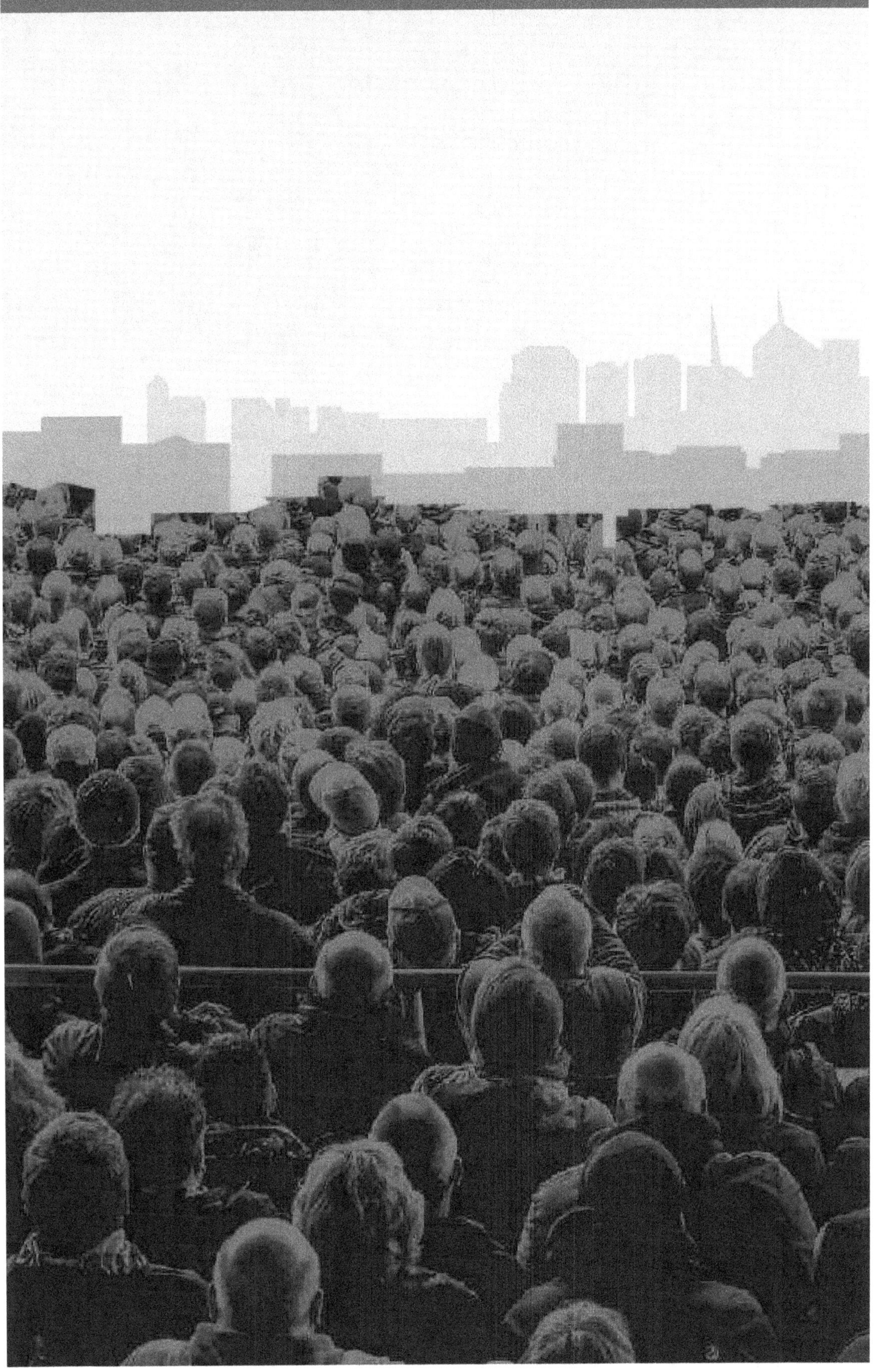

* 9 7 9 8 3 0 5 4 1 2 2 8 4 *